PICKLEBALL

chartwell
books

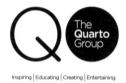

Inspiring | Educating | Creating | Entertaining

Brimming with creative inspiration, how-to projects, and useful information to enrich your everyday life, quarto.com is a favorite destination for those pursuing their interests and passions.

This edition published in 2023 by Chartwell Books,
an imprint of The Quarto Group
142 West 36th Street, 4th Floor
New York, NY 10018 USA
T (212) 779-4972 F (212) 779-6058
www.Quarto.com

10 9 8 7 6 5 4 3 2 1

Chartwell titles are also available at discount for retail, wholesale, promotional, and bulk purchase. For details, contact the Special Sales Manager by email at specialsales@quarto.com or by mail at The Quarto Group, Attn: Special Sales Manager, 100 Cummings Center Suite 265D, Beverly, MA 01915, USA.

ISBN: 978-0-7858-4206-4

Publisher: Wendy Friedman
Senior Managing Editor: Meredith Mennitt
Senior Design Manager: Michael Caputo
Editor: Joanne O'Sullivan
Designer: Kate Sinclair

All stock design elements ©Shutterstock

Printed in China

Game On!

If you've caught on to the joys, the challenges, and the undeniable appeal of pickleball, you're not alone! It's been the fastest growing sport in the US for nearly a decade and its popularity has begun to spread around the world. As the sport reaches new players, the level of play continues to rise, too. Pickleball is easy to learn but taking your game to the next level requires focus. Whether you're a newcomer to the sport or a more experienced player, you can improve your pickleball skills by applying game-specific strategies and tried-and-true methods for enhancing your mental focus.

Pickleball is known for being easier on the joints, knees, and elbows than tennis. While it may be gentler on the body, it requires mental agility. 'Getting your head in the game' is one of the most important steps you can take to invest in your pickleball skills.

If you've already tried pickleball, you know how addictive it can be. Beyond the rewards of game play, it's a social sport with a tight-knit and supportive community of players. Pickleball can be part of your life for years to come, so it's worth the time and effort to focus on your enhancing skills. That's what this book is for.

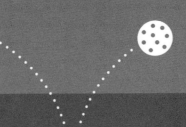

Improving Your Game

One of the reasons for pickleball's popularity is the simplicity of the game. It's easy to learn and players report being able to master the basics after a short time. But what about going beyond the basics? We've compiled some of the most useful tips from experienced pickleball players to help you up your game. In addition to skills-based techniques, we'll introduce you to useful insight on sports psychology so you can sharpen your mental game as well. With this powerful framework for thinking about the game, you'll be able to achieve the mind-body connection that will take you to the next level.

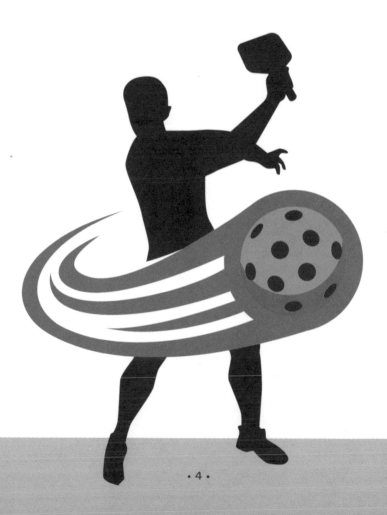

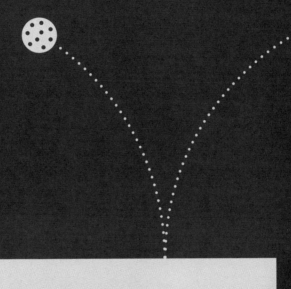

"Setting goals is the first step in turning
the invisible into the visible."

TONY ROBBINS

TRACKING YOUR PROGRESS

Why track your progress? Research shows that self-reflection and accountability are essential to self-improvement. That applies to all areas of life, from personal and professional goals to fitness. If you're reading this, you've decided to commit your time and attention in improving your pickleball game. For some, that might mean being able to play in a local tournament. For others, it might mean going even further.

You might invest in time with a trainer or a coach. Or you might try to create your own plan. You may want to do both. Start planning with this book. With tools, prompts, and exercises that help you to analyze your own performance, you'll be able to measure you own progress, pat yourself on the back, and keep moving toward your goals.

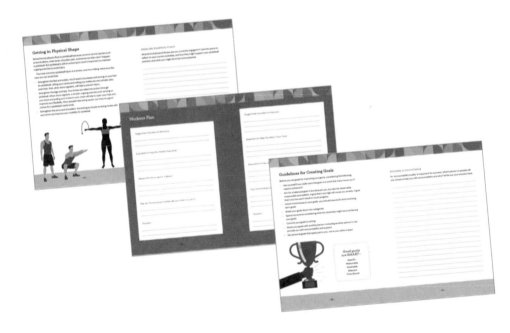

How to Use This Book

This book is designed to be used at your own pace. Whether your pickleball improvement journey takes three months or a year, you can still track your progress. The most important thing is to set goals that work with your own life and your own schedule. You can customize the tools to work with your own time frame.

We'll start with a quick review of pickleball history, vocabulary, game play, rules, and a few other basics. Then we'll move into aspects of training, both physical and mental. There's no prescribed workout plan or timeline for your reflections. Instead, the resources should be used as guides. If you decide, for example, that you hate squats and will never do a single one, that's ok. You can take the advice "you need to do warm ups" and tailor it to your own preferences. A flexible plan is one that you are more likely to stick with. A plan you stick with is one that points you toward success.

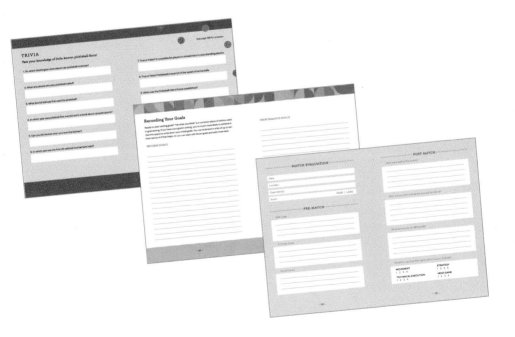

"Make sure your worst enemy doesn't
live between your own two ears."

LAIRD HAMILTON
professional surfer

ADJUST YOUR APPROACH

Are you a beginner at pickleball? You may have heard that it's incredibly easy to learn and play. Players who've caught pickleball fever tend to be very enthusiastic and love to recruit new players to join in the fun. But remember, even something that is considered easy by some is not easy for all. With any sport or game, there is a learning curve. If you stepped onto the court and found it more challenging than you thought it would be based on everything you've heard, you are not alone. It may be relatively easy compared to another activity or it may not be easy for you at all. That's ok!

When we consider something to be easy, we might think it doesn't require any effort. When it comes to learning a new sport, that's just not the case. It will take time. It will take effort. It's more than likely that you won't change to instantly be great at it.

Now is a good time to start thinking about your approach to pickleball. Even if you believe it to be easy, take your pathway to physical and mental fitness for the game seriously. An easy, fun game can also be a serious pastime!

Use this space to reflect upon what you think you know or what you believe about pickleball as you begin your improvement process.

ADJUST YOUR MINDSET

Have you heard the saying that 90 percent of sports performance is mental? It's a common bit of wisdom shared by coaches. It's also often ignored. But overlooking mental performance in a game is a mistake. And by putting effort into 'focusing on focus' and 'paying attention to your attention,' you'll be surprised at how this kind of mental training can really affect your game.

If you're accustomed to thinking of 'training' or preparation for a game as stretches and perhaps a jog, allow yourself to expand your thinking. Chances are that in other areas of your life, you set goals and then plot a path to achieving them—a big vacation requires planning; a new house requires savings. Why not apply this incremental, steady-progress-toward-a-goal mentality to your pickleball play? With milestones, check-in's, and trackers, you can achieve success with your game performance, too.

Use this space to reflect upon a time when you set goals, checked in on them regularly, and ultimately achieved them.

_____

_____

_____

_____

_____

_____

_____

_____

_____

Getting
Started

Ready for a little review? In this section of the book, we'll take a look at some of the history and basics of the sport. You can test yourself on trivia and knowledge of the game and prepare a pre-game fitness and skills plan.

What Do You Know About Pickleball?

A rainy day. Bored kids stuck indoors. A bunch of classic lake house sports equipment, including a wiffle ball and ping-pong paddles. Joel Pritchard, Bill Bell, and Barney McCallum had all these things on a summer afternoon in 1965 on Bainbridge Island, Washington. What they did with those things changed their lives. A game they created to keep the kids entertained turned into the sport of pickleball. First a game just for the men's immediate friends and family, pickleball spread with a slow burn over the course of decades.

Pickleball is a creative hybrid of different sports, often called "ping-pong on steroids." It's played indoors or outdoors on a court that is shorter than a tennis court, with a ball that's similar to a wiffle ball and a paddle that's a little like an oversize ping-pong paddle. There's a rumor that the game was named after Pritchard's dog Pickles, but McCallum said that it was actually named after the 'pickleboat' in rowing (a boat in which rowers use oars left over from other boats). His wife Joan said that the game reminded her of that particular situation—a sport made from equipment and strategies from other sports.

Since that rainy day in 1965, the sport has gained momentum with a speed that's surprised almost everyone. It was mostly a local backyard game in the Pacific Northwest until the early 1980s. Now there are around 35,000 courts in the US.

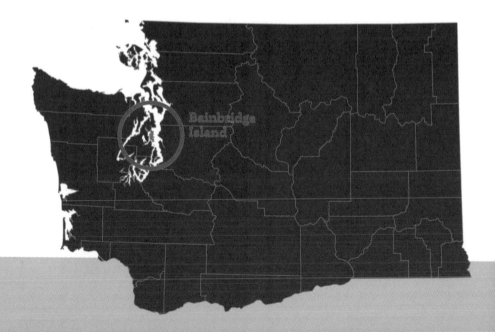

What is it about pickleball that's so enticing?

Players say it's easy to learn and easy on the knees and elbows, making it a great alternative to tennis, which can lead to injuries in these sensitive areas. Because the pickleball court is shorter than a tennis court, there's less running involved. The rules are simple, so the game is easy to learn and master in a short time.

There's a satisfying *pock* as the ball hits the paddle and sails across the net. The volley continues at a fast pace: there's no need for a lunge across the court, just a quick shift to meet the ball. This isn't tennis, it's pickleball and it's believed to be the fastest growing sports in the US.

Pickleball Today

The sport grew slowly through the first few decades after it was invented. It gained popularity throughout the Pacific Northwest throughout the late 60s and 1970s. You may be surprised to learn that Microsoft founder Bill Gates was an early adopter of the game. His father was a friend of the inventors of pickleball. Bill Gates, Sr. liked the game so much he even had a court built at the family home. So Bill, Jr. has been playing pickleball most of his life, and considers it one of his favorite sports.

Once the popularity of pickleball began to spread, it first caught on with seniors in retirement communities. While seniors are still the highest percentage of pickleball players, it's now played by people of all ages, and young and old can play the game together. Elementary, middle, and high schools have begun to offer pickleball as a school fitness option. In 2021, a major league pickleball league was formed and there is even an effort underway to make pickleball an Olympic sport.

If you are just now catching the pickleball bug, you're not too late. Now is a perfect time to get started in the sport. It's known to have a very welcoming community, and you'll find many who are ready to encourage you and offer tips and practice with you.

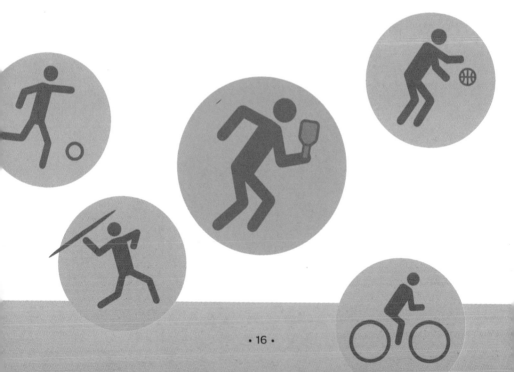

MY PICKLEBALL DISCOVERY STORY

Use this space to describe your first encounter with pickleball. How did you hear about it? Did you see people playing it and wonder what it was? Did you want to be part of a community? Challenge yourself? Both? Think about what makes you excited to commit to learning more.

TRIVIA

Test your knowledge of little-known pickleball facts!

1. On which Washington state island was pickleball invented?

2. What are people who play pickleball called?

3. What kind of ball was first used for pickleball?

4. In which year was pickleball first mentioned in a book about racquet sports?

5. Can you hit the ball when you're in the kitchen?

6. In which year was the first US national tournament held?

See page 188 for answers

7. True or False? It's possible for players in wheelchairs to play standing players.

8. True or False? Pickleballs travel 1/3 of the speed of tennis balls.

9. When was the Pickleball Hall of Fame established?

10. True or False? A pickleball can be any color.

11. Is pickleball going to be an Olympic sport?

12. What's the total size of a pickleball paddle?

Final Score: / 12

Pickleball Basics

Part of the appeal of pickleball is the simplicity of the game. You don't need to invest a lot to get started and you don't have to have a lot of experience or athletic ability. Let's look at a few things you need to know before stepping on the court.

THE EQUIPMENT

Pickleball equipment is simple! You only need the following.

A PADDLE Pickleball paddles come in different shapes, widths, and weights, and with different handles and grips. They are generally made out of wood, graphite (aluminum), or composite. It's a good idea to hold a paddle in your hand before you buy it rather than buying one online. You want to get one that feels right in your hand: not too heavy or light, with a comfortable grip. Beginners tend to start with a lighter paddle. In terms of the grip, many players determine the length according to their height. For players under 5'2", a 4-inch grip is recommended. Players over 5'2" should start with a 4.5-inch grip.

A BALL Pickleballs can be any color. There is a distinction between balls for indoor and outdoor play, but other than that, it's up to you.

NET If you want to practice at home, you can pick up a portable net.

CLOTHING You can wear anything you want to play pickleball! Most players wear tennis shoes in the style of their preference.

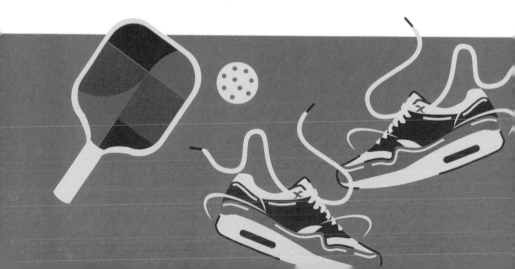

THE COURT

The pickleball court is 20 x 44 feet, with a center net measuring 36 inches high at the edges and 34 inches high at the center. You'll notice an important area on either side of the net—the non-volley zone, otherwise known as the kitchen.

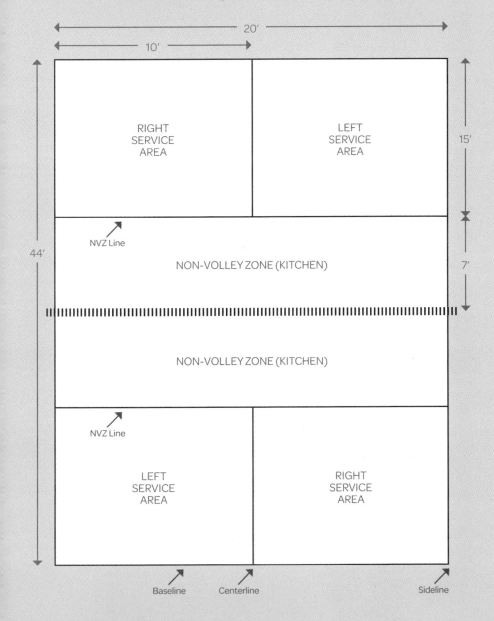

Basic Rules

While it's a little more complicated than this, you can boil down the basic rules of pickleball to these.

- Keep the ball in bounds. If you hit the ball out of bounds, you lose your serve.
- When you begin, the ball must bounce on serve and return, but only once per side. If you let the ball bounce twice on your side, you lose your turn, and the ball goes to the other team. After the initial volley, the two-bounce rule kicks in (see opposite page).
- You must serve from the baseline, with one foot behind it.
- Serve must be done underhand, ball held below the waistline, to the opponent at a diagonal to you across the net.
- The serve can't land in the 'non-volley zone,' or kitchen. When a volley is returned, it can enter that area (see opposite page).
- The game will end at 11 or 15 points. The winning score is 11, but the winning team must win by 2 points, so it's possible that the game will have to continue to 15 points.

Once you know these basic rules, you're ready to begin playing.

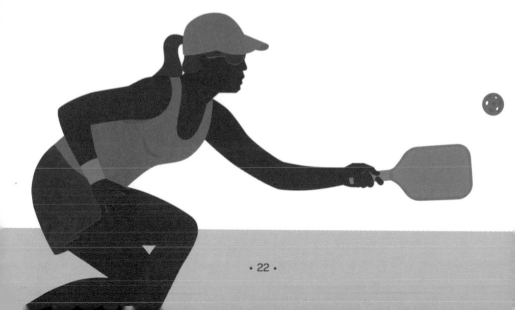

Beyond the Basics

- The right side always serves first. If a point is scored, the server changes sides and starts the next serve from the left side. As additional points are scored, the server continues switching sides until a fault is committed and the first server loses the serve.

- When the first server loses the serve, their partner then serves from their correct side of the court. The second server continues serving until his team commits a fault and loses the serve to the opposing team.

- At the start of the game, the serving team can have only one fault (see page 27) before giving up the serve to their opponent. (A fault is a violation of a rule that stops play. Faults must be tallied throughout the game.) After that, both members of each team will serve until two team faults have been committed before turning the ball over to the opponent.

- Both players on the serving doubles team can serve and score points until they commit a fault (except for the first service sequence of each new game).

- In singles, the server serves from the right-hand side when their score is even and from the left when the score is odd.

The Double-Bounce Rule

Each team must play their first shot off the bounce. That means the receiving team must let the serve bounce before returning it and the serving team must let the return bounce before hitting it back. After that, all balls can be volleyed or returned off a bounce.

The Serve

The serve is central to pickleball play. Here are a few basics to know about serves.

- Serves must come from behind the baseline and serves must be underhand, from below the waist. Both the volley and return must happen within a 10-second time frame. Once the score has been called, you've got 10 seconds to serve. If you don't get the serve out in 10 seconds, you get a fault.
- Beyond that, rules vary a little depending on whether you're playing singles or doubles.

SINGLES

Players serve until they lose a point. Players must switch the side they're serving from after each serve. If your score is even, you serve from the right side of the court. If your score is odd, serve from the left. When you call out the score, call your own score, then your opponent's score.

DOUBLES

At the start of a new game, only one player serves before play passes to the other team. After that, each player on the team has the opportunity to serve before the serve passes to the other team.

KINDS OF SERVES OR SHOTS

POWER SERVE This is one of the most popular serves in pickleball, served low and hard toward the back of the court, aimed at getting your opponent in a defensive position.

VOLLEY SHOT Hit with a powerful punch, it's usually aimed down the non-volley line.

DINKING/DROP SHOT Aimed to arch over the net and land in the kitchen/non-volley zone, it's a good choice when the opponent is near the back at the baseline.

KITCHEN CORNER SERVE This serve is aimed to land just outside the opponent's kitchen. It's a light, strategic serve.

LOB SERVE Also known as the High Soft Serve or the Moon Ball Serve, this is a high-arching serve sent at a slow to medium pace, intended to land near the baseline.

CENTERLINE SERVE This serve is a bit advanced and a bit tricky. It involves leaning toward the centerline as you serve and aiming the ball toward the opponent's center line with the goal of causing it to bounce.

OVERHEAD SMASH (OR SPIKE) This shot is a powerful one, hit hard down the non-volley/kitchen line.

DRIVE SHOT This is a line drive or straight shot.

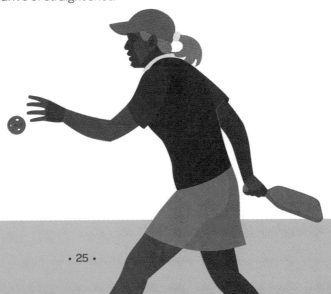

Scoring and Faults

The team that goes first is determined by a coin toss.

DOUBLES SCORING

- Points are scored only from serving. Receiving players can't score a point.
- Game play starts on the right. If a point is scored, the server moves to the left side and continues to serve diagonally across the court.
- The serving team continues to move from the right to left or left to right each time a point is scored, but only if a point is scored. The receiving team doesn't switch sides.
- The first server continues to serve until the serving team commits a fault.
- When the second server loses the serve, the serve goes to the other team and the player on the right serves first throughout the game.
- A score is called in this sequence: server score, receiver score, then, for doubles only, the server number: 1 or 2. At the beginning of the match, the score is zero - zero – two to indicate the second server.

SINGLES SCORING

Singles scoring is very similar to doubles except that there is no second server. The serve is always from the right when the server's score is even and from the left on odd. The server's score determines the serving position, not the score of the receiver. The receiver lines up on the right or left side according to the server's score. The score is called server score, receiver score.

FAULTS

Players are given a fault when:

- They hit the ball out of bounds
- The ball doesn't clear the net
- They step in the non-volley zone/kitchen and volley the ball
- They volley the ball before it has bounced once on each side of the net
- They hit the ball into the net
- They don't return the ball before it bounces twice
- Any part of the player, including their clothing or paddle, touches the net when the ball is in play
- The ball in play hits any part of the player (except if the ball touches below the wrist of the player's paddle hand)
- The ball is hit before it passes the plane of the net
- A ball hits the post.

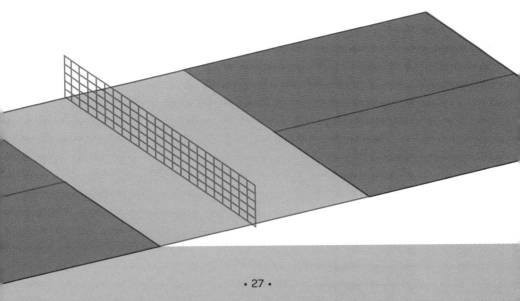

Score Sheet

Use these sample score sheets, adapted from official score sheets developed by USA Pickleball, to practice scoring.

MATCH WINNER SCORES

Game 1 _____/_____ Game 2 _____/_____ Game 3 _____/_____ Initials_____

SERVE	SCORE																						TIME OUTS
S	1 2 3 4 5 6 7 8 9 10 11 12 13 14 15 16 17 18 19 20 21																						1 2 3
S	1 2 3 4 5 6 7 8 9 10 11 12 13 14 15 16 17 18 19 20 21																						1 2 3
S	1 2 3 4 5 6 7 8 9 10 11 12 13 14 15 16 17 18 19 20 21																						1 2 3

MATCH WINNER SCORES

Game 1 _____/_____ Game 2 _____/_____ Game 3 _____/_____ Initials_____

SERVE	SCORE																						TIME OUTS
S	1 2 3 4 5 6 7 8 9 10 11 12 13 14 15 16 17 18 19 20 21																						1 2 3
S	1 2 3 4 5 6 7 8 9 10 11 12 13 14 15 16 17 18 19 20 21																						1 2 3
S	1 2 3 4 5 6 7 8 9 10 11 12 13 14 15 16 17 18 19 20 21																						1 2 3

MATCH WINNER SCORES

Game 1 _____/_____ Game 2 _____/_____ Game 3 _____/_____ Initials_____

SERVE	SCORE																						TIME OUTS
S	1 2 3 4 5 6 7 8 9 10 11 12 13 14 15 16 17 18 19 20 21																						1 2 3
S	1 2 3 4 5 6 7 8 9 10 11 12 13 14 15 16 17 18 19 20 21																						1 2 3
S	1 2 3 4 5 6 7 8 9 10 11 12 13 14 15 16 17 18 19 20 21																						1 2 3

MATCH WINNER SCORES

Game 1 _____/_____ Game 2 _____/_____ Game 3 _____/_____ Initials_____

SERVE	SCORE	TIME OUTS
S	1 2 3 4 5 6 7 8 9 10 11 12 13 14 15 16 17 18 19 20 21	1 2 3
S	1 2 3 4 5 6 7 8 9 10 11 12 13 14 15 16 17 18 19 20 21	1 2 3
S	1 2 3 4 5 6 7 8 9 10 11 12 13 14 15 16 17 18 19 20 21	1 2 3

MATCH WINNER SCORES

Game 1 _____/_____ Game 2 _____/_____ Game 3 _____/_____ Initials_____

SERVE	SCORE	TIME OUTS
S	1 2 3 4 5 6 7 8 9 10 11 12 13 14 15 16 17 18 19 20 21	1 2 3
S	1 2 3 4 5 6 7 8 9 10 11 12 13 14 15 16 17 18 19 20 21	1 2 3
S	1 2 3 4 5 6 7 8 9 10 11 12 13 14 15 16 17 18 19 20 21	1 2 3

MATCH WINNER SCORES

Game 1 _____/_____ Game 2 _____/_____ Game 3 _____/_____ Initials_____

SERVE	SCORE	TIME OUTS
S	1 2 3 4 5 6 7 8 9 10 11 12 13 14 15 16 17 18 19 20 21	1 2 3
S	1 2 3 4 5 6 7 8 9 10 11 12 13 14 15 16 17 18 19 20 21	1 2 3
S	1 2 3 4 5 6 7 8 9 10 11 12 13 14 15 16 17 18 19 20 21	1 2 3

Vocabulary

ACE A serve that is not returned by the opposing team

BACKCOURT The area around the baseline

BASELINE The line at the back of the court, 22 feet from the pickleball net

CENTERLINE The dividing line that separates the service court into halves from the non-volley zone to the baseline

CROSS-COURT DINK A dink that carries all the way from one side of the court to the other and usually lands in the opposite opponent's kitchen

FAULT/ERROR A point lost because of mistakes (see page 27)

FOOT FAULT When the server fails to keep one foot behind the line

HALF VOLLEY A shot where a ball bounces but doesn't reach full height before it is hit

LET A point that must be replayed

LET SERVE A serve that hits the top of the net but otherwise is legal. Must be re-served

LINE CALL A statement that determines whether a ball is in or out

NON-VOLLEY ZONE Also called the kitchen. The 7-foot-area surrounding the net into which players can't step until the ball has bounced or, on follow-through, until the ball is down. Serves must clear this area to be considered good

POACH When players take shots going to their partners. Poaching often takes place when the skill of the team members is mismatched.

PUNCH A quick shot with a minimal backswing, similar in motion to stabbing the ball out of the air with the paddle

PUT AWAY A shot that the opponent cannot return, therefore a winning shot

RALLY Continuous play after a serve

SERVER NUMBER If playing doubles, the server must call their number – either "one" or "two," based on who serves first or second on their side. This number must be called out along with the score

TOP SPIN A shot with spin caused by hitting the ball with the paddle swinging from low to high. Some pickleball players buy a pickleball paddle for spin specifically

SKINNY SINGLES A game played with two people, one on each side, using only half of the court

VOLLEY A ball hit before it bounces

Pickleball Slang

FLAPJACK A shot that must bounce once before it can be hit

"PICKLE!" The word that players shout when then are about to serve

PICKLED When a team doesn't score any points

PICKLEDOME A court where a pickleball championship is played

PICKLER A slang term for pickleball players

"The two things you are in control of in your life are your attitude and your effort."

ANONYMOUS

QUIZ

1. Which three sports is pickleball based on?

2. Who were the three founders of pickleball?

3. In what year was pickleball invented?

4. What size is a pickleball court?

5. How high is a pickleball net?

6. What is the name for the seven-foot area surrounding the net?

See page 190 for answers.

7. True or False? A point can be earned only by the serving team.

8. True or False? You'll get a fault if you step in the non-volley zone to volley.

9. What score wins a pickleball game?

10. How long is an average pickleball match?

11. True or False? Pickleball is considered to be the fastest-growing sport in the US.

12. What is a dink shot?

Final Score: / 12

My Pickleball Questions

As you're learning about pickleball, you'll probably have questions about a lot of things, from rules to strategies to scoring. Use this space to write down questions that come up. You can do your own research or ask a friend or trainer. Keep this page bookmarked or use a sticky note so you can return to it and add questions as you continue to learn!

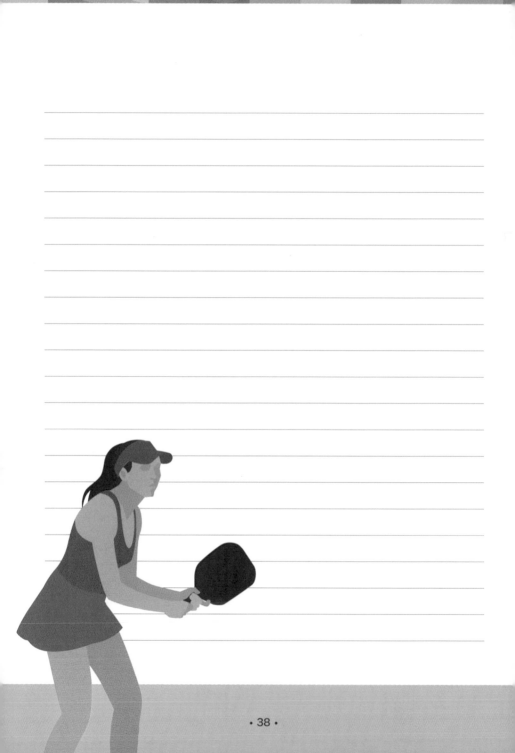

Getting in Physical Shape

Retired tennis players flock to pickleball because common tennis injuries such as tennis elbow, wrist strain, shoulder pain, and tennis toe often don't happen in pickleball. But pickleball is still an active sport and it's important to maintain ongoing exercise to avoid injury.

The most common pickleball injury is a broken wrist from falling. Here are a few ways you can avoid that.

- Strengthen the feet and ankles. You'll need to be steady and strong on your feet for pickleball. Lifting your calves and rolling your ankles are very simple, easy exercises, that, when done regularly, will help to prevent injury.
- Strengthen the legs and hips. Your knees are called into action through pickleball. When done regularly, a simple, ongoing exercise such as lying on your back and pulling your knees to your chest will help to open your hips and improve your flexibility. Many people hate doing squats, but they're a good choice for a pickleball-ready body.
- Strengthen the arms and shoulders. Something as simple as doing circles with your arms can improve your mobility for pickleball.

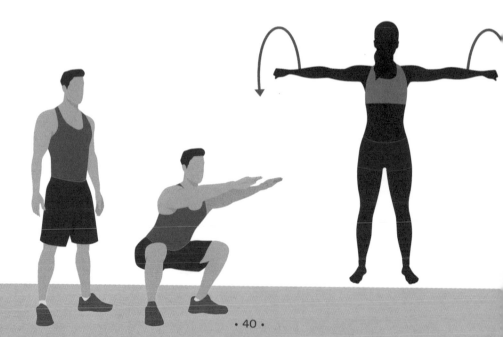

EXERCISE STARTING POINT

What kind of physical fitness are you currently engaged in? Use this space to reflect on your current activities, and how they might support your pickleball practice, and what you might do to be more prepared.

Warm-Ups

Even though pickleball is easy to learn and easy on the body, it's important to warm up before practice or matches. Warming up goes a long way toward preventing injuries. You should also work on getting your heart rate going and warming up your muscles before play.

You can ask your club members or friends which exercises work best for them, but here are a few ideas to get you started. Plan on warming up for at least 10 minutes before each match.

- March in place, getting your knees up. Swing your arms as you do it.
- Run the length of the court several times.
- Raise your knees and twist to each side.
- Raise your knees and try to touch elbow to opposite knee.
- Do a series of arm circles.
- Practice lunges across the court.
- Do a series of squats.

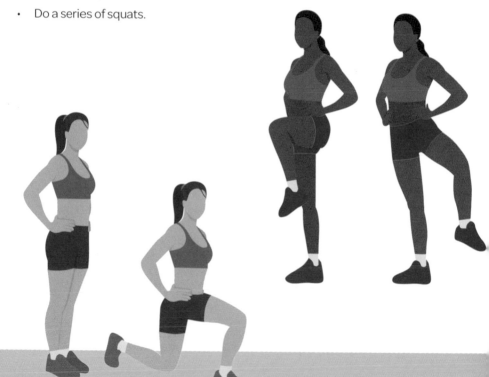

SELF-EVALUATION

Have you incorporated warm-ups into your sports practice in the past? What works best for you? Do you prefer to warm up alone or with others? Use this space to articulate your viewpoint on warm-ups and what you think you can commit to doing in order to improve at pickleball.

Drills

It may seem basic and repetitive, but doing drills will build your muscle memory and help you go into your matches with confidence. Drills aren't as fun as actually playing the game, but they'll go a long way toward helping you master ball control and more.

- Wall drill: Practice your forehand and backhand technique by hitting the ball against a wall.
- Dinking for points: Practice hitting the ball to only one side of the court
- Triangle dinking: Hit the ball to three different points of the court in a prescribed sequence.
- Back-and-forth drill: Start at the kitchen line and dink the ball to a partner who is also standing at the kitchen line. Your partner should step back and return the ball. Each player will step back each time they hit the ball until they reach the baseline.

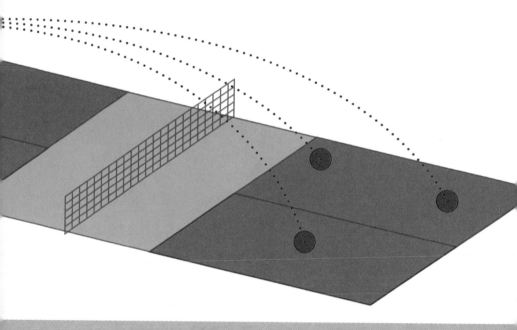

"If you only ever give 90 percent in training, then you will only ever give 90 percent when it matters."

MICHAEL OWEN

SELF-EVALUATION

Use this space to express your commitment to a training routine. Consider time, space, and availability of training partner.

_____

_____

_____

_____

_____

_____

YOUR PICKLEBALL ROLE MODEL

Do you have a pickleball player you look up to? Someone you'd like to use as a role model for your pickleball play? Write about that player and what you admire about their play. This could be someone you know, someone in your local club, or a famous player. What is it about their play that you'd like to emulate?

_____

_____

_____

_____

_____

_____

YOU AS A TEAM MEMBER

More often than not, you'll be playing doubles pickleball, so you will be part of a team. What is your experience working with a team or as a partner? Use this space to reflect upon your experience with team sports. What role do you usually take? Are you a leader or more of a supporter? How is playing pickleball with a partner the same or different than playing singles? What would you like to do differently in your pickleball play as a doubles partner?

Cooldowns

It's tempting to skip cooling down after pickleball, but it's an important step in preventing injuries, stiffness, and soreness. Leg cramps are among the most common types of pickleball injuries (along with broken wrists). Spending just a little time cooling down can help ensure you're not sidelined. Here are some helpful cool down steps to take.

- Jog down the court a couple of times at an easy pace.
- Do a few sides steps.
- Stretch those quads. Grab the toe of your shoe with the opposite hand behind your back and hold for about 10 seconds while balancing on your other leg. Do the same with your other foot.
- Bend and reach toward your toes with a flat back and legs apart. Hold for around 10 seconds.
- Give yourself a hug: stretch your arm across your chest, over your shoulder and hold until you feel the stretch.
- Do a slow walk around the court.

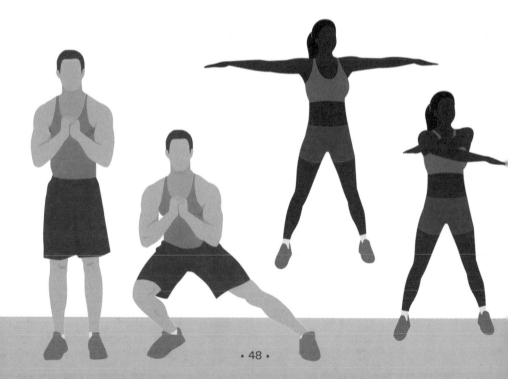

SELF EVALUATION

Sure, it' tempting to skip off for a cool beverage after a match, but taking those few extra minutes will really help. Use this space to think about your post-match patterns: are you eager to socialize? Want to replay the game in your head? Use this space to record your post-game routines and think about how you can work in time for a cool down.

"Success is where preparation
and opportunity meet."

BOBBY UNSER

Developing a Training Plan

Use this space to develop a training plan for different aspects of your play. Think about your different resources, what you're willing to and motivated to do, and who might help you.

Workout Plan

Target Area You Want to Improve

_____

_____

Exercises to Help You Reach Your Goal

_____

_____

_____

Resources (time, space, trainer)

_____

_____

_____

Plan for Development (what will you commit to do?)

_____

_____

Timeline

_____

_____

Target Area You Want to Improve

_____

_____

_____

Exercises to Help You Reach Your Goal

_____

_____

_____

Resources (time, space, trainer)

_____

_____

_____

Plan for Development (what will you commit to do?)

_____

_____

_____

Timeline

_____

_____

Drills Practice

What skills do you need to improve?

_____

_____

What drills will help you?

_____

_____

_____

Resources (time, space, partner)

_____

_____

_____

What drills can you commit to doing regularly?

_____

_____

_____

Timeline

_____

_____

What skills do you need to improve?

_____

_____

_____

What drills will help you?

_____

_____

_____

Resources (time, space, partner)

_____

_____

_____

What drills can you commit to regularly doing?

_____

_____

_____

Timeline

_____

_____

Drills Practice

What skills do you need to improve?

_____

_____

What drills will help you?

_____

_____

_____

Resources (time, space, partner)

_____

_____

_____

What drills can you commit to doing regularly?

_____

_____

_____

Timeline

_____

_____

What skills do you need to improve?

_____

_____

_____

What drills will help you?

_____

_____

_____

Resources (time, space, partner)

_____

_____

_____

What drills can you commit to regularly doing?

_____

_____

_____

Timeline

_____

_____

Individual Skills Practice

What skills do you need to improve?

_____

_____

_____

_____

_____

How will you train to get better?

_____

_____

_____

_____

_____

_____

Resources

_____

_____

_____

DON'T FORGET TO HAVE FUN!

While getting your mind and body in shape for pickleball is a serious pursuit, don't lose sight of a very important factor in pickleball's overwhelming popularity—it's fun! Use this space to reflect upon what's fun about pickleball for you or perhaps to tell a story about some of the fun experiences you've had playing the game. Fun can be a very motivating factor!

QUIZ

1. Which side always serves first?

2. Is a ball that lands on the line still good?

3. By how many points must the winner win?

4. At the beginning of a game, how many faults is the serving team allowed before they have to give up their serve?

5. Once the play progresses, how many faults is the serving team allowed?

6. What is a lob?

See pages 191 for answers

7. What is a foot fault?

8. What is a rally?

9. What is a 'let'?

10. True or False? A player, the player's paddle or clothing must not touch the net.

11. What is a drop shot?

12. What is the double-bounce rule?

Final Score: / 12

TRIVIA

Test your knowledge of little-known pickleball facts!

1. In which year was pickleball invented?

2. How many holes are there in a pickleball?

3. How high is a pickleball net?

4. In which year was USA Pickleball formed?

5. Around how many pickleball courts are there in the US?

6. Around how many people play pickleball in the US?

See page 189 for answers

7. In which year did pickleball become the official state sport of the state of Washington?

8. Around how many professional pickleball teams are there?

9. What city is considered the pickleball capital of the world?

10. What is the word for what happens when a team scores zero points in a game? The team is_____.

11. True or False? There is a major league pickleball organization.

12. True or False? The average age for pickleball players is 38.

Final Score: _____ / 12

Getting Your Head in the Game

Now that you've spent some time developing a plan for physical training, turn toward your mental game. It's equally, if not more, important than your physical fitness. Having a strong 'head game' can help you to stay focused, which will, in turn, improve your skills on the court.

Where I'm Starting From

In order to track your progress, you'll need to pinpoint your starting line. Think about your current situation with pickleball. Use these two pages to document the beginning of your journey. Knowing your baseline measurement will make it easier later to see how far you've come! Some points you might cover: How serious do you currently feel about your pickleball practice? What role does pickleball currently play in your life? You may want to include some reflection on your experience and success with other sports versus how you feel about your current level in pickleball.

Skills Inventory

Take an honest look at where you are with your skills and evaluate yourself. This table is based on an assessment developed by USA Pickleball. Rate yourself on a scale of one to five. Use these guidelines to help you determine your rating. Check the box next to the level you think applies to you.

☐ **LEVEL 1.0**
• Absolute beginner, completely new to the game

☐ **LEVEL 1.5**
• Actively pursuing lessons
• Learning rules
• Learning how to serve
• Developing a forehand

☐ **LEVEL 2.0**
• Beginning to develop skills
• Can maneuver around the court to a degree
• Understands where to stand during play and how to serve and receive
• Gets some serves in
• Knows how to keep score

LEVEL 2.5

- Increasing skill at serving
- Starting to dink
- Improving form on ground strokes
- Can lob with forehand
- Improving court coverage

LEVEL 3.0

- Improved ability to play as a team member
- More powerful shots
- Starting to lob and dink
- Improved shot strokes and shot placement

LEVEL 3.5

- Deeply understands the rules of the game
- Gets most serves "in"
- Can serve and return serve deep
- Can determine opponent's weaknesses
- Exercises strategic game play
- Works well with partner
- Hits fewer balls out of bounds

LEVEL 4.0

- Anticipates opponents' moves
- Plays mostly offensively
- Plays strategically
- Varies shots to create a competitive advantage
- Works well with partner and easily switches court positions
- Can block volleys
- Good footwork
- Few unforced errors

LEVEL 4.5

- Calm, confident play
- High level of strategy
- Quick, controlled movement
- Sustained volleys
- Excellent placement of shots
- Ability to adjust style of play and game plan according to opponents' strength and weaknesses and court position

LEVEL 5.0

- Has mastered all skills and strategies
- Keeps calm and focused
- Fast, agile, and athletic

"Remember: sports are
meant to be fun."

A.J. KITT
US World Cup skier

Your Starting Point

SHOT SKILLS

Here's another way to think about your starting point. Circle the number that best describes your experience.

5	You don't have to think about a shot before taking it and you're still successful.
4.5	You don't have to think about taking a shot, but you also don't always hit successfully.
4	You have to think about a shot, and when you figure it out, you are successful.
3.5	You have to think about a shot, and you aren't always successful.
3	You overthink your shots, so you're too late to hit them.
1-2	You just hit randomly and don't make many shots.

SERVES

Give yourself a score of one to five (or half measures) on these different types of pickleball serves. Write the number next to the type of serve.

	Power Serve
	Centerline Serve
	Kitchen Corner Serve
	Spin Serve

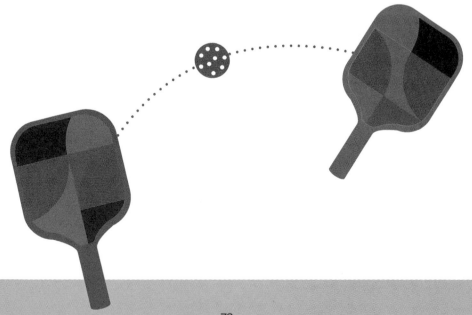

Your Starting Point

STRATEGY SKILLS

Check the box next to the statement that most closely resembles your level.

	I don't know much about the strategy of the game. I'm at the point where I'm just trying to get the ball back over the net.
	I'm learning about strategy and aiming my shots more strategically, but I don't have a wide variety of shots yet.
	I know a number of shots now. I'm starting to get the hang of when to use them.
	I make a point of matching my shots to the situation.
	I enjoy studying strategy and applying it as I play.

FOOTWORK SKILLS

Check the box next to the statement that most closely resembles your level.

	I miss shots because I'm not fast enough yet.
	My ability to anticipate where a shot will land is improving.
	I can quickly determine where a shot will land and get there in time.
	I'm able to move around the court quickly to keep play going successfully.
	I'm always or almost always in the right place at the right time.

COMMUNICATION SKILLS

Check the box next to the statement that most closely resembles your level.

	The only way I speak to my partner is to say yours, mine, or out.
	I am starting to communicate observations with my partner during the game.
	I communicate directions to my partner.
	I communicate a lot with my partner and we move together as a team.
	My partner and I play as a unit.

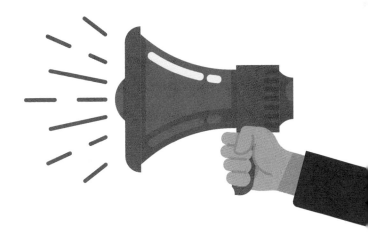

What's My Motivation?

What makes you truly successful at your pursuits? You may seek a community or personal achievement. You may be looking to find a long-term outlet that will help you stay fit. You may just be looking for a challenge. Think about what motivates you to improve your pickleball practice, using these prompts to help you.

- Think about a time when you were highly motivated. Write it down.
- Think about a time you were demoralized. Write it down.
- Identify aspects of your personality that might affect your motivation, such as "I'm competitive," "I love learning new skills," or "Sports are social for me." List these characteristics below.

PICKLEBALL PRIORITIES

Use the space below to record your motivations for improving your pickleball practice. Rank them in order of priority.

During your week days, notice what kind of activities get you excited and motivated. What made your day good or bad? Try to link your positive moods to motivations. If you like, ask your teammates or club members what motivates them!

Why Do You Love Pickleball?

Take some time to think about why you are interested in improving your pickleball game. You'll be most successful if you're doing something you love. Consider some of these aspects of the game that might motivate you:

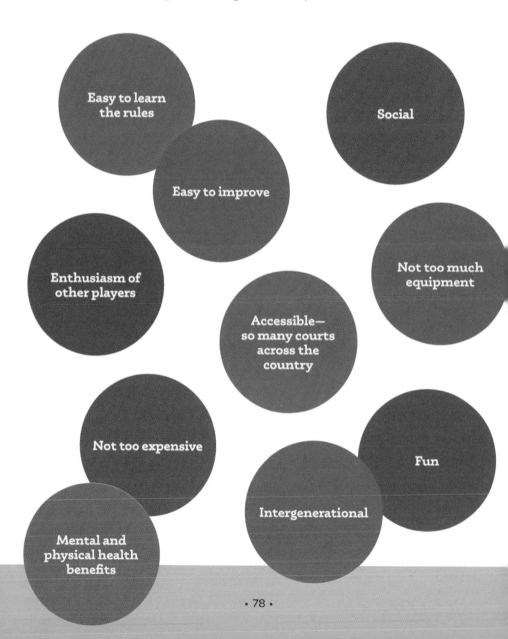

Easy to learn the rules

Social

Easy to improve

Enthusiasm of other players

Not too much equipment

Accessible— so many courts across the country

Not too expensive

Fun

Intergenerational

Mental and physical health benefits

I HEART PICKLEBALL

Use this space to write out the reasons you're drawn to the game and why you are invested in getting better at it.

Establishing Goals for Your Game

You're here because you want to improve your game. Research shows that articulating and committing to goals goes a long way toward success and achievement.

Start with being very specific and intentional about what you want to achieve. That word specific is important. But what exactly does that mean? Not all goals are created equal.

A goal that is too vague decreases your chance for success. "Get better" or "Do my best" doesn't push you far enough.

In deciding what you want to achieve, it might help to look at different types of goals. Think of these three types: process goals, performance goals, and outcome goals. When you're working on your pickleball performance, you can break down your goals in these categories.

THE THREE TYPES OF GOALS

PROCESS GOALS A process goal is about the actions you take. For example, if you decide that you will practice a certain skill for 15 minutes, three times a week, that's a process goal. This type of goal is a commitment that you set and you control.

PERFORMANCE GOALS This kind of goal is about a standard that you hold yourself to. For example, if you want to set a goal that you will score a certain number of points per game, or steadily increase the number of points you score over the course of a time period. While you can't control it completely, it gives you a standard to work toward.

OUTCOME GOALS This is your end goal. For example, if you want to qualify for a tournament or achieve a certain ranking in your pickleball league. It might be simpler, such as "I will master an excellent serve." Outcome goals are not entirely within your control.

In addition to these three types of goals, you may wish to specifically think about teamwork goals.

"The great danger for most of us lies not in setting our aim too high and falling short, but in setting our aim too low and achieving our mark."

MICHELANGELO

Guidelines for Creating Goals

Before you set goals for improving your game, considering the following:

- Ask yourself if you really want this goal–is it worth the many hours you'll need to achieve it?
- Aim for a balanced goal: it should push you, but also be observable, measurable and realistic. A goal that's too high will cause you anxiety. A goal that's too low won't result in much progress
- Attach time frames to your goals–you should have both short and long-term goals
- Break your goals down into categories
- Spend some time considering what the obstacles might be to achieving your goals
- Commit your goals to writing
- Share your goals with another person–including another person in can provide you with accountability and support
- Set personal goals that apply just to you, not to you within a team

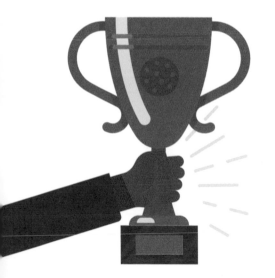

Good goals are SMART—

Specific,
Measurable,
Attainable,
Relevant
Time-Bound

STAYING ACCOUNTABLE

An 'accountability buddy' is important for success. Which person or people will you chose to help you with accountability and why? Write out your answers here.

Recording Your Goals

Ready to start setting goals? "Ink what you think" is a common piece of advice used in goal setting. If you have your goal in writing, you're much more likely to achieve it. Use this space to write down your initial goals. You can brainstorm a list of up to ten then narrow it if that helps. Or you can start with fewer goals and add more later.

PROCESS GOALS

PERFORMANCE GOALS

OUTCOME GOALS

TEAMWORK GOALS

Visualize Your Success

Visualization can be a powerful way to help you achieve your goals. Studies show that imagining your 'best self' is proven to help you achieve the progress you desire.

Take a moment to picture what it will be like when you overcome the gap between where you are now in your game practice. What does your success look like? Where are you when you realize you've been successful? Be specific—what are you wearing? Who are you with? What's the weather like? Describe the scene using all five senses. Don't edit or judge yourself. Give yourself 10 minutes to record the scene in writing here.

_____

_____

_____

_____

_____

_____

Write a Vision Statement

Write a vision statement that summarizes where you want to be when you finish. Keep it somewhere you can see it as an ongoing reminder!

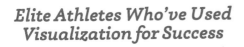

Elite Athletes Who've Used Visualization for Success

- Rock climber Alex Honnold
- NBA star LeBron James
- Olympic swimmer Michael Phelps
- Olympic diver Greg Louganis

> "Visualization is daydreaming with a purpose."
>
> BO BENNETT

Action Plans

An action plan can help you achieve your goals. If provides clarity, outlines tasks, and helps you to focus both your attention and your resources. Spend some recording your action plans on the pages that follow.

Goal

_____

_____

Plan to reach goal

_____

_____

_____

Tasks associated with goal

_____

_____

_____

Reflection

_____

_____

_____

Goal

_____

_____

_____

Plan to reach goal

_____

_____

_____

_____

_____

Tasks associated with goal

_____

_____

_____

_____

Reflection

_____

_____

_____

_____

Goal

_____

_____

_____

Plan to reach goal

_____

_____

_____

_____

Tasks associated with goal

_____

_____

_____

_____

Reflection

_____

_____

_____

_____

Goal

_____
_____
_____

Plan to reach goal

_____
_____
_____
_____
_____

Tasks associated with goal

_____
_____
_____
_____

Reflection

_____
_____
_____
_____

Goal

_____

_____

_____

Plan to reach goal

_____

_____

_____

_____

_____

Tasks associated with goal

_____

_____

_____

_____

Reflection

_____

_____

_____

_____

"The trouble with not having a goal is that you can spend your life running up and down the field and never score."

BILL COPELAND

Goal-Setting Timeline

Add your goals and time markers to the timeline.

GOAL	TIMELINE FOR ACHIEVEMENT

GOAL	TIMELINE FOR ACHIEVEMENT

GOAL	TIMELINE FOR ACHIEVEMENT

GOAL	TIMELINE FOR ACHIEVEMENT

GOAL	TIMELINE FOR ACHIEVEMENT

GOAL	TIMELINE FOR ACHIEVEMENT

Calming Your Anxiety

Staying on track requires calming your anxiety. So, how do you do that? Here are some tips:

- Focus on the now. Staying in the moment is the secret of the best athletes. Try not to get ahead of yourself.
- Train yourself to recognize when your focus is shifting.
- Comparing yourself to others is a sure-fire way to lose focus and amp up your anxiety. No matter what any of the other players are doing, you are only responsible for you.
- Remember, pickleball is supposed to be fun. Keeping enjoyment in mind will have benefits that affect all aspects of your game play. It will help you to take the pressure off yourself.
- Don't overthink it. Imagine you've spent a lot of time training for a match. When you step on to the court, your mind gets in a whirl trying to remember it all. Slow down. If you've really prepared, your training will kick in. Opening your mind is better than clamping down on the steps you need to remember.
- Remember that there are many variables you can't control. When you begin to focus on something outside your control, you'll lose attention on those things that you can.

List it Out

By anticipating the mental traps you may fall into, you can avoid them. Take a few moments to examine your game play and determine what aspects of your play you can control and which you can't.

Things I Can Control in My Game

_____

_____

_____

_____

_____

_____

_____

_____

_____

_____

_____

_____

_____

Things I Can't Control

_____

_____

_____

_____

_____

_____

_____

_____

_____

_____

_____

_____

_____

Being in the Moment

You step out onto the court to start a game. What's the first thing that comes to your mind? Is it your last disastrous game? Or wanting this game to be over? When you're thinking of the past or the future, you're not aligned with the action on the court. You're also stressing yourself out. Practicing mindfulness will:

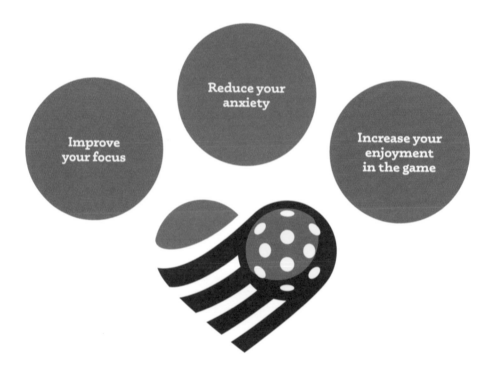

Improve your focus

Reduce your anxiety

Increase your enjoyment in the game

TO PRACTICE AT HOME

- Focus on your breathing. Sit with your eyes closed. Breathe in deeply and slowly. Hold your breath. Exhale slowly. Repeat this process at least five times. Try to make it a daily practice.

- Do a 'body scan.' While in sitting position or lying on your back, start at your feet and feel the sensation in each part of your body, from your toes upward. This will raise your awareness of your body and help you stay centered. Try doing this daily.

- Notice your breath and body together.

- Try 'noticing' your thoughts without judgement. They are thoughts, not truths. They will come and go like the weather. When you have a negative thought, recognize it as just that: a thought that will pass and not necessarily true.

DURING YOUR MATCH

- Decide where to place your focus: your breathing? The ball as it touches your opponent's paddle? Practice focusing on one thing and see what results you get.

- Create a simple ritual. Maybe you hop before you serve or return. Maybe you touch your shoe. Focusing on your ritual will help prevent you from thinking negative thoughts.

- Notice your thoughts. If you're distracted, bring yourself back to your breathing.

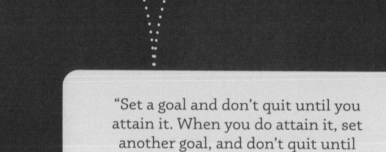

"Set a goal and don't quit until you attain it. When you do attain it, set another goal, and don't quit until you reach it. Never quit."

BEAR BRYANT

Positive Self Talk

While you're training for the physical demands and strategies of your game, you may consider training your mind as an afterthought. But it's an important part of your process. You may not always feel confident about your game, but it's important to believe that you can do it.

NEGATIVE SELF TALK	POSITIVE SELF TALK
I can't do this.	This is a chance to learn something new.
I don't have the time.	This is important to me. I'll prioritize it.
Everyone is better than me.	Right now, I'm just competing against myself.
I'm too uncoordinated.	Once I improve, I'll be able to sync my skills.
I should just be naturally good at this.	Everyone has to practice to improve.
I don't see enough progress.	Improvement takes time.

Inner Critic or Inner Coach

Who wins out when you are trying to master a new skill—your inner critic or your inner coach? Your inner critic replays everything you've done wrong in the past. This critic won't let go of past mistakes. But what about your inner coach? Your inner coach will tell you to keep going, that you can and will achieve your goals. Imagine what both your inner critic and inner coach would say to you about your current goals.

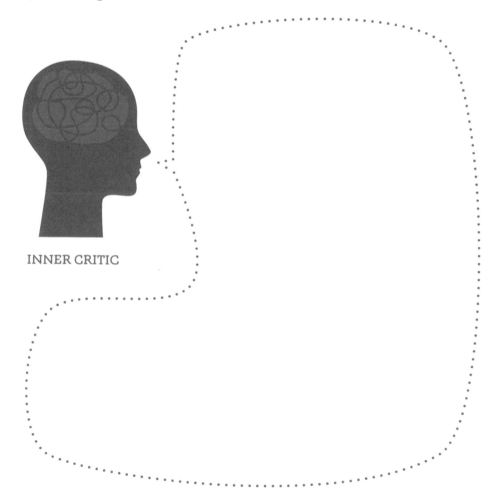

INNER CRITIC

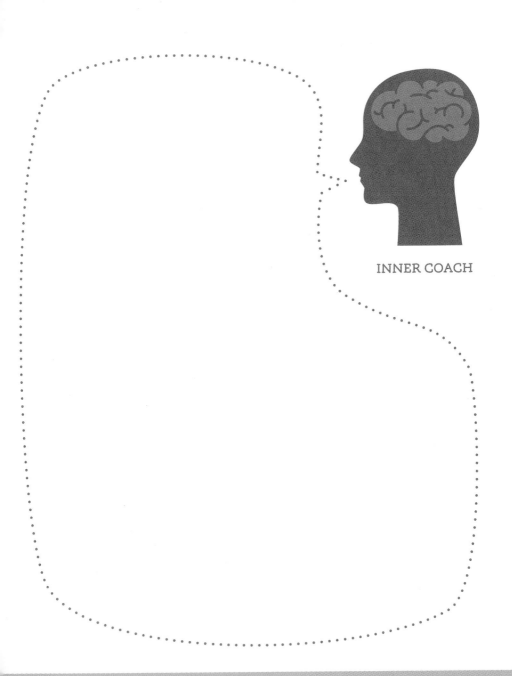

INNER COACH

Potential Obstacles

Trying to identify what might prevent you from reaching your goals helps you to anticipate roadblocks and plan for them. Imagine what might get in the way of your improvement, such as not having enough time, family commitments, fear, insecurity or a physical limitation. Then, think about how you might overcome that obstacle in order to continue with your progress.

POTENTIAL OBSTACLE

HOW I'LL OVERCOME IT

Affirmations

Repeating affirmations is a great way to introduce positive self-talk into your training routine. Here are some examples of affirmations you might use:

I am confident in my ability.
I enjoy the training process.
I am highly motivated to achieve my goals.
I can stay focused under pressure.
I can perform well in tough competitions.
I feel mentally strong.
I can stay positive throughout competition.
I like the challenge of competition.

I am a good hitter and have a variety of shots .
I have a strong serve that I can place where I want.
I enjoy practicing hard.
Through practice, I will achieve my athletic potential.
My stamina is always increasing.
I will push myself to become the best athlete in my sport.
I am dedicated and excited to practice.
I will meet and surpass my own expectations.

Affirmations—Try it Yourself

Use this space to create affirmations specific to your goals and your practice.

High Fives!

Accomplishments, no matter how small, should be celebrated! Use this space to pat yourself on the back. Be generous with yourself the way a coach or teammate would be.

Game
Tracking

We live in a data-driven world. Data is constantly being collected to improve products and services. Can you use it to improve your game? In this section of the book, you can track your performance across 30 games. Tracking will help you to focus on your improvements and identify areas that continue to pose challenges for you. Accountability is an important part of your success, even if (or especially if) you are accountable only to yourself.

MATCH EVALUATION

Date

Location

Opponent(s)

Score   WIN / LOSS

PRE-MATCH

Skill Goals

Strategy Goals

Mental Goals

What went well in this match?

What are you proud of about your performance?

What would you do differently?

Rank how you feel the match went (1=poor, 4=great)

MOVEMENT
1 2 3 4

STRATEGY
1 2 3 4

TECHNICAL EXECUTION
1 2 3 4

HEAD GAME
1 2 3 4

MATCH EVALUATION

Date

Location

Opponent(s)

Score   WIN / LOSS

PRE-MATCH

Skill Goals

Strategy Goals

Mental Goals

What went well in this match?

What are you proud of about your performance?

What would you do differently?

Rank how you feel the match went (1=poor, 4=great)

MOVEMENT
1 2 3 4

STRATEGY
1 2 3 4

TECHNICAL EXECUTION
1 2 3 4

HEAD GAME
1 2 3 4

··············· MATCH EVALUATION ···············

Date

Location

Opponent(s)

Score   WIN / LOSS

··················· PRE-MATCH ···················

Skill Goals

Strategy Goals

Mental Goals

What went well in this match?

What are you proud of about your performance?

What would you do differently?

Rank how you feel the match went (1=poor, 4=great)

MOVEMENT
1 2 3 4

STRATEGY
1 2 3 4

TECHNICAL EXECUTION
1 2 3 4

HEAD GAME
1 2 3 4

MATCH EVALUATION

Date

Location

Opponent(s)

Score   WIN / LOSS

PRE-MATCH

Skill Goals

Strategy Goals

Mental Goals

What went well in this match?

What are you proud of about your performance?

What would you do differently?

Rank how you feel the match went (1=poor, 4=great)

MOVEMENT
1 2 3 4

STRATEGY
1 2 3 4

TECHNICAL EXECUTION
1 2 3 4

HEAD GAME
1 2 3 4

MATCH EVALUATION

Date

Location

Opponent(s)

Score   WIN / LOSS

PRE-MATCH

Skill Goals

Strategy Goals

Mental Goals

What went well in this match?

What are you proud of about your performance?

What would you do differently?

Rank how you feel the match went (1=poor, 4=great)

MOVEMENT
1 2 3 4

TECHNICAL EXECUTION
1 2 3 4

STRATEGY
1 2 3 4

HEAD GAME
1 2 3 4

MATCH EVALUATION

Date

Location

Opponent(s)

Score   WIN / LOSS

PRE-MATCH

Skill Goals

_____

_____

_____

Strategy Goals

_____

_____

_____

Mental Goals

_____

_____

_____

What went well in this match?

What are you proud of about your performance?

What would you do differently?

Rank how you feel the match went (1=poor, 4=great)

MOVEMENT
1 2 3 4

STRATEGY
1 2 3 4

TECHNICAL EXECUTION
1 2 3 4

HEAD GAME
1 2 3 4

MATCH EVALUATION

Date

Location

Opponent(s)

Score   WIN / LOSS

PRE-MATCH

Skill Goals

Strategy Goals

Mental Goals

What went well in this match?

What are you proud of about your performance?

What would you do differently?

Rank how you feel the match went (1=poor, 4=great)

MOVEMENT
1 2 3 4

STRATEGY
1 2 3 4

TECHNICAL EXECUTION
1 2 3 4

HEAD GAME
1 2 3 4

Date

Location

Opponent(s)

Score	WIN / LOSS

······· **PRE-MATCH** ·······

Skill Goals

Strategy Goals

Mental Goals

What went well in this match?

What are you proud of about your performance?

What would you do differently?

Rank how you feel the match went (1=poor, 4=great)

MOVEMENT
1 2 3 4

STRATEGY
1 2 3 4

TECHNICAL EXECUTION
1 2 3 4

HEAD GAME
1 2 3 4

·············· MATCH EVALUATION ··············

Date

Location

Opponent(s)

Score   WIN / LOSS

···················· PRE-MATCH ····················

Skill Goals

Strategy Goals

Mental Goals

What went well in this match?

What are you proud of about your performance?

What would you do differently?

Rank how you feel the match went (1=poor, 4=great)

MOVEMENT
1 2 3 4

STRATEGY
1 2 3 4

TECHNICAL EXECUTION
1 2 3 4

HEAD GAME
1 2 3 4

Date

Location

Opponent(s)

Score   WIN / LOSS

•••••••••••••••••••••PRE-MATCH•••••••••••••••••••••

Skill Goals

Strategy Goals

Mental Goals

What went well in this match?

What are you proud of about your performance?

What would you do differently?

Rank how you feel the match went (1=poor, 4=great)

MOVEMENT
1 2 3 4

STRATEGY
1 2 3 4

TECHNICAL EXECUTION
1 2 3 4

HEAD GAME
1 2 3 4

MATCH EVALUATION

Date

Location

Opponent(s)

Score   WIN / LOSS

PRE-MATCH

Skill Goals

Strategy Goals

Mental Goals

What went well in this match?

What are you proud of about your performance?

What would you do differently?

Rank how you feel the match went (1=poor, 4=great)

MOVEMENT
1 2 3 4

STRATEGY
1 2 3 4

TECHNICAL EXECUTION
1 2 3 4

HEAD GAME
1 2 3 4

MATCH EVALUATION

Date

Location

Opponent(s)

Score   WIN / LOSS

PRE-MATCH

Skill Goals

Strategy Goals

Mental Goals

What went well in this match?

What are you proud of about your performance?

What would you do differently?

Rank how you feel the match went (1=poor, 4=great)

MOVEMENT
1 2 3 4

STRATEGY
1 2 3 4

TECHNICAL EXECUTION
1 2 3 4

HEAD GAME
1 2 3 4

Date

Location

Opponent(s)

Score   WIN / LOSS

····················· PRE-MATCH ····················

Skill Goals

Strategy Goals

Mental Goals

What went well in this match?

What are you proud of about your performance?

What would you do differently?

Rank how you feel the match went (1=poor, 4=great)

MOVEMENT
1 2 3 4

STRATEGY
1 2 3 4

TECHNICAL EXECUTION
1 2 3 4

HEAD GAME
1 2 3 4

MATCH EVALUATION

Date

Location

Opponent(s)

Score   WIN / LOSS

PRE-MATCH

Skill Goals

Strategy Goals

Mental Goals

What went well in this match?

What are you proud of about your performance?

What would you do differently?

Rank how you feel the match went (1=poor, 4=great)

MOVEMENT
1 2 3 4

STRATEGY
1 2 3 4

TECHNICAL EXECUTION
1 2 3 4

HEAD GAME
1 2 3 4

Date

Location

Opponent(s)

Score   WIN / LOSS

· PRE-MATCH ·

Skill Goals

Strategy Goals

Mental Goals

What went well in this match?

What are you proud of about your performance?

What would you do differently?

Rank how you feel the match went (1=poor, 4=great)

MOVEMENT
1 2 3 4

STRATEGY
1 2 3 4

TECHNICAL EXECUTION
1 2 3 4

HEAD GAME
1 2 3 4

MATCH EVALUATION

Date

Location

Opponent(s)

Score   WIN / LOSS

PRE-MATCH

Skill Goals

Strategy Goals

Mental Goals

What went well in this match?

What are you proud of about your performance?

What would you do differently?

Rank how you feel the match went (1=poor, 4=great)

MOVEMENT
1 2 3 4

STRATEGY
1 2 3 4

TECHNICAL EXECUTION
1 2 3 4

HEAD GAME
1 2 3 4

MATCH EVALUATION

Date

Location

Opponent(s)

Score   WIN / LOSS

PRE-MATCH

Skill Goals

Strategy Goals

Mental Goals

What went well in this match?

What are you proud of about your performance?

What would you do differently?

Rank how you feel the match went (1=poor, 4=great)

MOVEMENT
1 2 3 4

STRATEGY
1 2 3 4

TECHNICAL EXECUTION
1 2 3 4

HEAD GAME
1 2 3 4

Date

Location

Opponent(s)

Score   WIN / LOSS

················ PRE-MATCH ················

Skill Goals

Strategy Goals

Mental Goals

What went well in this match?

What are you proud of about your performance?

What would you do differently?

Rank how you feel the match went (1=poor, 4=great)

MOVEMENT
1 2 3 4

TECHNICAL EXECUTION
1 2 3 4

STRATEGY
1 2 3 4

HEAD GAME
1 2 3 4

·············· MATCH EVALUATION ···············

Date

Location

Opponent(s)

Score   WIN / LOSS

····················· PRE-MATCH ·····················

Skill Goals

Strategy Goals

Mental Goals

What went well in this match?

What are you proud of about your performance?

What would you do differently?

Rank how you feel the match went (1=poor, 4=great)

MOVEMENT
1 2 3 4

STRATEGY
1 2 3 4

TECHNICAL EXECUTION
1 2 3 4

HEAD GAME
1 2 3 4

MATCH EVALUATION

Date

Location

Opponent(s)

Score   WIN / LOSS

PRE-MATCH

Skill Goals

Strategy Goals

Mental Goals

What went well in this match?

What are you proud of about your performance?

What would you do differently?

Rank how you feel the match went (1=poor, 4=great)

MOVEMENT
1 2 3 4

STRATEGY
1 2 3 4

TECHNICAL EXECUTION
1 2 3 4

HEAD GAME
1 2 3 4

Date

Location

Opponent(s)

Score | WIN / LOSS

Skill Goals

Strategy Goals

Mental Goals

What went well in this match?

What are you proud of about your performance?

What would you do differently?

Rank how you feel the match went (1=poor, 4=great)

MOVEMENT
1 2 3 4

STRATEGY
1 2 3 4

TECHNICAL EXECUTION
1 2 3 4

HEAD GAME
1 2 3 4

MATCH EVALUATION

Date

Location

Opponent(s)

Score   WIN / LOSS

PRE-MATCH

Skill Goals

Strategy Goals

Mental Goals

What went well in this match?

What are you proud of about your performance?

What would you do differently?

Rank how you feel the match went (1=poor, 4=great)

MOVEMENT
1 2 3 4

STRATEGY
1 2 3 4

TECHNICAL EXECUTION
1 2 3 4

HEAD GAME
1 2 3 4

MATCH EVALUATION

Date

Location

Opponent(s)

Score   WIN / LOSS

PRE-MATCH

Skill Goals

Strategy Goals

Mental Goals

What went well in this match?

What are you proud of about your performance?

What would you do differently?

Rank how you feel the match went (1=poor, 4=great)

MOVEMENT
1 2 3 4

STRATEGY
1 2 3 4

TECHNICAL EXECUTION
1 2 3 4

HEAD GAME
1 2 3 4

MATCH EVALUATION

Date

Location

Opponent(s)

Score   WIN / LOSS

PRE-MATCH

Skill Goals

Strategy Goals

Mental Goals

What went well in this match?

What are you proud of about your performance?

What would you do differently?

Rank how you feel the match went (1=poor, 4=great)

MOVEMENT
1 2 3 4

STRATEGY
1 2 3 4

TECHNICAL EXECUTION
1 2 3 4

HEAD GAME
1 2 3 4

·············· MATCH EVALUATION ··············

Date

Location

Opponent(s)

Score   WIN / LOSS

·················· PRE-MATCH ··················

Skill Goals

_____
_____
_____

Strategy Goals

_____
_____
_____

Mental Goals

_____
_____
_____

What went well in this match?

What are you proud of about your performance?

What would you do differently?

Rank how you feel the match went (1=poor, 4=great)

MOVEMENT
1 2 3 4

STRATEGY
1 2 3 4

TECHNICAL EXECUTION
1 2 3 4

HEAD GAME
1 2 3 4

MATCH EVALUATION

Date

Location

Opponent(s)

Score   WIN / LOSS

PRE-MATCH

Skill Goals

Strategy Goals

Mental Goals

What went well in this match?

What are you proud of about your performance?

What would you do differently?

Rank how you feel the match went (1=poor, 4=great)

MOVEMENT
1 2 3 4

STRATEGY
1 2 3 4

TECHNICAL EXECUTION
1 2 3 4

HEAD GAME
1 2 3 4

Date

Location

Opponent(s)

Score   WIN / LOSS

················· PRE-MATCH ·····················

Skill Goals

Strategy Goals

Mental Goals

What went well in this match?

What are you proud of about your performance?

What would you do differently?

Rank how you feel the match went (1=poor, 4=great)

MOVEMENT
1 2 3 4

STRATEGY
1 2 3 4

TECHNICAL EXECUTION
1 2 3 4

HEAD GAME
1 2 3 4

MATCH EVALUATION

Date

Location

Opponent(s)

Score   WIN / LOSS

PRE-MATCH

Skill Goals

Strategy Goals

Mental Goals

What went well in this match?

What are you proud of about your performance?

What would you do differently?

Rank how you feel the match went (1=poor, 4=great)

MOVEMENT
1 2 3 4

STRATEGY
1 2 3 4

TECHNICAL EXECUTION
1 2 3 4

HEAD GAME
1 2 3 4

Date

Location

Opponent(s)

Score   WIN / LOSS

···················· PRE-MATCH ·····················

Skill Goals

Strategy Goals

Mental Goals

What went well in this match?

What are you proud of about your performance?

What would you do differently?

Rank how you feel the match went (1=poor, 4=great)

MOVEMENT
1 2 3 4

STRATEGY
1 2 3 4

TECHNICAL EXECUTION
1 2 3 4

HEAD GAME
1 2 3 4

MATCH EVALUATION

Date

Location

Opponent(s)

Score   WIN / LOSS

PRE-MATCH

Skill Goals

Strategy Goals

Mental Goals

What went well in this match?

What are you proud of about your performance?

What would you do differently?

Rank how you feel the match went (1=poor, 4=great)

MOVEMENT
1 2 3 4

STRATEGY
1 2 3 4

TECHNICAL EXECUTION
1 2 3 4

HEAD GAME
1 2 3 4

What I Learned

Now that you've tracked your games, use this space to record your observations. Try to sum up what you've learned about your skills, areas for improvement, and new goals for the future.

_____

_____

_____

_____

_____

_____

_____

_____

_____

_____

_____

_____

_____

_____

_____

_____

_____

_____

_____

_____

_____

What I Learned

"You dream. You plan. You reach. There will be obstacles. There will be doubters. There will be mistakes. But with hard work, with belief, with confidence and trust in yourself and those around you, there are no limits."

MICHAEL PHELPS

What I Learned

TRIVIA ANSWERS

Answers to trivia questions on pages 18-19

1. On which Washington state island was pickleball invented?
   Bainbridge Island

2. What are people who play pickleball called?
   Picklers

3. What kind of ball was first used for pickleball?
   A wiffle ball

4. In which year was pickleball first mentioned in a book about racquet sports?
   1978

5. Can you hit the ball when you're in the kitchen?
   No

6. In which year was the first pickleball national championship held?
   2009

7. True or False? It's possible for players in wheelchairs to play standing players.
   True

8. True or False? Pickleballs travel 1/3 of the speed of tennis balls.
   True

9. When was the Pickleball Hall of Fame established?
   2017

10. True or False? A pickleball can be any color.
    True

11. Is pickleball going to be an Olympic sport?
    It's not yet, but there is a movement to have it included.

12. What's the total size of a pickleball paddle?
    24 inches total, 16 inches long, 8 inches wide.

Answers to trivia questions on pages 62-63

1. In which year was pickleball invented?
   1965

2. How many holes are there in a pickleball?
   Most outdoor pickleballs have 40 holes while most indoor pickleballs have 26.

3. How high is a pickleball net?
   36 inches on the side and 34 in the center

4. In which year was USA Pickleball formed?
   2005

5. Around how many pickleball courts are there in the US?
   Around 35,000

6. Around how many people play pickleball in the US?
   Around 4.8 million

7. In which year did pickleball become the official state sport of the state of Washington?
   2022

8. Around how many professional pickleball teams are there?
   The are 12 teams in the major league pickleball association.

9. What city is considered the pickleball capital of the world?
   Naples, Florida

10. What is the word for what happens when a team scores zero points in a game? The team is_____.
    Pickled

11. True or False? There is a major league pickleball organization.
    True

12. True or False? The average age for pickleball players is 38.
    True

QUIZ ANSWERS

Answers to quiz questions on pages 34-35

1. Which three sports is pickleball based on?
   Badminton, wiffle ball, and ping pong

2. Who were the three founders of pickleball?
   Joel Pritchard, Bill Bell, and Barney McCallum

3. In what year was pickleball invented?
   1965

4. What size is a pickleball court?
   20 x 44 feet

5. How high is a pickleball net?
   36 inches high on the ends and 34 in the center

6. What is the name for the seven-foot area surrounding the net?
   The non-volley zone or kitchen

7. True or False? A point can be earned only by the serving team.
   True

8. True or False? You'll get a fault if you step in the non-volley zone to volley.
   True

9. What score wins a pickleball game?
   11 or 15

10. How long is an average pickleball match?
    Between 15 and 25 minutes

11. True or False? Pickleball is considered to be the fastest-growing sport in the US.
    True

12. What is a dink shot?
    A soft shot that arcs and lands in the opponent's kitchen

Answers to quiz questions on pages 60-61

1. Which side always serves first?
   The right side

2. Is a ball that lands on the line still good?
   Yes

3. By how many points must the winner win?
   Two

4. At the beginning of a game, how many faults is the serving team allowed before they have to give up their serve?
   One

5. Once the play progresses, how many faults is the serving team allowed?
   Two

6. What is a lob?
   A high arching shot that lands near the baseline of the opponent.

7. What is a foot fault?
   When the server fails to keep a foot behind the line when serving

8. What is a rally?
   Continuous play after a serve.

9. What is a 'let'?
   A serve that hits the top of the net but otherwise is legal. Must be re-served

10. True or False? A player, the player's paddle or clothing must not touch the net.
    True

11. What is a drop shot?
    A ball hit that just clears the net and lands very close to the net in the non-volley zone.

12. What is the double-bounce rule?
    The double-bounce rule means the receiving team must let the serve bounce before returning it. The serving team must let the return bounce before hitting it back. After that, all balls can be volleyed or returned off the bounce.

Final Thoughts

What's next for your pickleball game? Use this space to determine your possible new goals now that you've documented your progress.

"If you are not willing to learn, no one can help you. If you are determined to learn, no one can stop you."

ZIG ZIGLAR